Introduct

If you want to apply for a place on an undergraduate Medicine course in the UK, but have no idea where to begin, I've written this book for you! I'm a Medical Student in the UK and I got offers for all four of my university choices. But, the journey to success wasn't easy!

I applied for Medical Schools when I was in year 13, and I got 1 interview and zero offers. I was so unprepared, baffled, and intimidated by the application process, I wasn't at all surprised to receive no offers. But I was determined to try again, so I took a gap year.

Between having my first set of applications rejected, and attending interviews for my new applications, nearly a year later, I learned so much about the application process. I felt so confident and prepared that I had a really strong feeling that I was going to get a place that year!

And that's how I want you to feel during the application process! So here is all my advice for getting into Medical School in the UK, as an undergraduate. I hope you find it useful!

Work Experience

Work experience is such an important part of the medical school application for a number of reasons.

1. It is your first opportunity to explore the medical world and decide if you actually want to pursue a career in medicine.

2. It gives you opportunities to improve skills that medical schools want you to demonstrate.
3. It provides you with valuable and authentic experiences to reflect on in your personal statement and interviews.

How to find Work Experience

Most universities like you to have work experience in places where you'll come into contact with doctors; so the best options are generally hospitals and GP surgeries. Getting work experience in these places can be a little tricky as a lot of places can't offer work experience, and the ones that can, sometimes have waiting lists. But don't let this deter you! You will be successful as long as you are persistent!

I got work experience at a GP surgery by emailing the practice managers of every single GP Surgery in my town. I got a whole load of rejections but one GP surgery said they could take me on; and one is all you need!

I found that the best way to get work experience is to ask everyone and anyone you can think of. Ask people that you know have done some work experience, how they went about finding it; ask your friends and family if they know anyone that works in the medical field that might be able to get you a placement; email departments at your local hospitals and ask if you can do some work experience there. If you ask as many people as possible, you are bound to hear a "yes" at some point.

Also, do some research; you might find that your town or county has a work experience programme for aspiring medics, which you can apply for.

*

Although the general advice around finding work experience is "it's about quality, not quantity", I would still advise you to get as much and as varied work experience as you can. The reason for this is; the more you expose yourself to the medical environment, the more awareness you will have about what it's really like, and the more mature and insightful you will come across in your personal statement and interviews. The first year I applied for medical school, I had done 2 days of work experience in A&E and I thought I knew from that, exactly what A&E was like. Little did I know, I had been present for two of the quietest and most uneventful days the A&E department had ever seen, and so in my personal statement and interview, I had nothing very profound to express, other than an unrealistic perception of A&E. It was only when I got a job at the same A&E department, as a Healthcare Assistant, during my gap year, that I realised how little insight I had the first time I applied for medical school. It was only when I worked the twelve-and-a-half-hour day and night shifts; properly interacted with and cared for patients; experienced the stress of a hospital at full capacity; became part of a real team of doctors and nurses, that I understood the reality of A&E.

Now, I am not at all saying that you need to work as a healthcare assistant for a year to get the insight you need to get into medical school, because this is not the case. What I am saying is; take every opportunity you get to enter the medical world, because the more you do, the more you will understand and appreciate what it is really like.

*

How to get the most out of your Work Experience

It isn't possible for everyone to get tonnes and tonnes of work experience, so I have some advice for you on how you can make the most of your work experience, so you can get the insight you need to impress universities.

Always have a notebook and pen on you so that you can take notes about what you are seeing, and what you have learned from that experience. If you're not allowed to carry a notebook, have one in your bag so that during your lunch break or at the end of the day, you can make notes about what you've seen while it's still fresh in your mind. Try to make your notes as comprehensive as possible and think about all the ways a case can help you understand and appreciate concepts in the medical world. It's not so much about documenting as many cases as possible; it's more about documenting a few good cases that give you lots to reflect on.

Here is an example of the sort of notes you could make on your work experience:

Work experience day 1; A&E Department

Male patient, aged 77 brought in by ambulance after a fall at home.

Doctor reads notes before seeing patient. From notes she sees patient has dementia and lives alone.

Doctor examines patient and asks questions like "Who is the current prime minister?" to assess his dementia. She examines the patient to look for injury. Patient's right leg is turned out and shorter than the left - indicates a fractured neck of femur. She sends patient for x-ray.

Patient was confused during examination - doctor says it's due to dementia. Doctor spoke simply and clearly to patient, repeating herself when patient didn't understand. This taught me the importance of being able to adapt your manor and approach to a patient, based on their needs.

Doctor called patient's daughter in to discuss care the patient receives at home, daughter says he has carers visit him twice a week. From patient's past medical history, doctor sees the patient has had a few falls recently. Doctor talks with daughter about getting patient more care and possibility of a care home to prevent any further injuries.

This taught me the importance of a holistic approach to patient care, because just dealing with the leg fracture meant the patient could fall and hurt themselves again once back home, but now things will be put in place to keep the patient safe.

This case has also shown me the importance of community care in reducing pressure on hospitals, because the more community care is given to those in need, the less people will sustain injuries that need treating in hospital.

Ask as many questions as you can to as many people as you can. This will help you get a real understanding of how the department, ward, GP surgery etc. that you are in, works and will help you get some context for what you are seeing and experiencing. If there is anything you don't understand; ask. If you see a staff member and you can't work out what their job is, ask someone. If you don't understand why a doctor asked a patient a certain question, ask them.

Some examples of good questions to ask might be:

What do you do within your role? – Helps you understand and appreciate the roles and responsibilities of different healthcare disciplines.

What do you think could be done better here? – It's great to get the opinion of someone that experiences the problems of a department on a daily basis, as they probably have great ideas about ways to improve the NHS (which is a topic that comes up in interviews from time to time).

Do you like your role? – Helps you gauge how people feel about their job and the NHS; whether people feel under too much pressure or responsibility, or whether they think things are doing smoothly for them.

Do you think patients are happy here? – a weird question as patient's generally aren't happy to be poorly and in a healthcare setting, but what this question is really getting at is, are patients receiving good quality of care. This can lead you on to finding out what is going well, to achieve good quality of care, and what needs to be improved to make care better. As well as asking staff this question, you could even ask patients how they feel about their care, if an appropriate opportunity arises.

Is this what it's usually like here? – Helps you gauge whether you've come on an abnormally quiet or busy day, so you can picture what kind of experience is had by patients and staff, generally.

Don't just focus on what doctors are doing. It's important to have an appreciation for the healthcare setting as a whole, which includes a lot more roles than just doctors. It will really help your insight if you can understand and appreciate the roles of other healthcare professionals (such as nurses, healthcare assistants, pharmacists, occupational therapists etc.) and what they do for patients, as well as what they do to allow doctors to better carry out their role. It is important on your work experience that you understand that doctors are not the most important members of the multidisciplinary team; nor are they "the bosses" of the team. They work alongside other healthcare professionals to achieve the shared goal of providing patients with high quality care. So look out for situations during your work experience that demonstrate this; it could be something useful to reflect upon in your personal statement or during your interviews.

Look for examples of good patient experiences and bad patient experiences. These will help you reflect on what actually went on; what skills were used well or not so well, to lead to a certain outcome for a patient.

A good patient experience might allow you to reflect on a doctor's good practice. For example, if a patient feels calm and reassured about a diagnosis they have recently received, you could reflect on the way that the doctor explained the diagnosis to the patient. Perhaps they explained the diagnosis, and what will happen next, clearly, calmly and thoroughly; spoke with a friendly, polite, and reassuring manor; asked if the patient had any questions etc.

A bad patient experience might allow you to reflect on an important skill that could have been used better. For example, a patient might be feeling frustrated because they have been forced to postpone an important scan, as they didn't know the scan required patients to have a full bladder, so they attended their scan with an empty bladder. Perhaps, you could reflect on the fact that communication between the doctor and the patient wasn't as good as it could have been. Maybe the doctor rushed through the explanation of the scan; used complicated medical terminology as if they were speaking to a colleague rather than a patient; and didn't ask the patient if they had any questions.

When it comes to patient experiences, it is always important to reflect on exactly what a situation means for the patient.

Something that may seem of little significance to you or even to a healthcare professional, may have a much more profound effect on the patient. For example, at first glance, it may seem minor that a healthcare assistant told a patient they would bring them some jam for their toast, and then forgot to do so. But, a patient that has been in hospital for many weeks, feeling extremely unwell and low in mood, who is struggling with weakness due to their lack of appetite; may be extremely disheartened and hurt by the fact that when they finally fancied some jam on toast and thought they might be able to get some strength back, they were forgotten about. In healthcare setting, each and every action a member of staff makes, no matter how tiny, can have a huge impact on a patient. Therefore, the responsibility each staff member carries is huge. It is so important to never forget the responsibility you hold as a healthcare worker, no matter your specific role. The effect of any action on a patient should always be at the forefront of your mind; it is something that is very important to reflect on, not only because it shows universities that you have a very developed sense of empathy and responsibility, but because a good doctor always thinks of the patient first.

*

Volunteering

Another great form of work experience, which you can do on top of your GP or hospital placements, is volunteering. Volunteering is great because it allows you to demonstrate long term commitment to something, as well as responsibility and organisation, by being able to balance your studies with voluntary work. Volunteering can also help to demonstrate benevolence and altruism as you are giving up your time for free to the community. What's more is that long term volunteering will give you the chance to develop lots of key skills such as empathy, people skills, organisation, time management, problem solving, and more, that will prepare you for not only, medical school interviews, but more importantly, life as a doctor. There are lots of volunteering opportunities out there; have a look online for voluntary work in your area. You could work in a charity shop; become a St John Ambulance Cadet; help out at your local hospital, hospice, primary school, youth club, care home; the possibilities are endless.

Like with GP or hospital work experience, it is a good idea to make notes about any experience that you have learned from. For example, when I volunteered at my local hospice, I found that I really improved my people skills and empathy. In the first few weeks I was quite shy, and I didn't know what to say to the patients or their families. But as the weeks went on, I gained more confidence, and observed how the nurses interacted with patients. I learned how to interact with patients to make them as comfortable as possible; I could read their body language and facial expressions a lot better, so that I could work out whether a light hearted conversation would make them feel a little brighter, or if they wanted to be alone.

Even if your volunteering doesn't relate directly to medicine, there are so many skills to be developed, that you can harness as a doctor. Let's say you volunteered in a primary school, and another volunteer was off sick for a number of weeks, so your workload doubled. This could be a great opportunity to develop your time management skills and your ability to cope under pressure.

Personal Statement

The personal statement is a short essay about you and your experiences, and why those things make you suitable for medicine. It's your first opportunity to show universities why you'd be a good doctor, other than the fact that you're academically able.

Some medical schools put more emphasis on the personal statement than others; a few universities barley look at the personal statement, if at all. But at the very least, a personal statement can be used as a 'tie-breaker'. If a medical school has two borderline candidates and they want to decide who, out of the two, to offer a place to, they might look at the personal statements to see who they think is the more appropriate choice. Therefore, no matter which medical schools you apply to, it is a very good idea to put a decent amount of time and effort into writing and polishing your personal statement.

Some people will have a finished personal statement in two or three drafts; others will take 15-20 drafts to get to a version they are happy with. It's a very individual thing so don't worry if people you know have had a very different 'personal statement journey' to you. The advice I will give you, though, is don't get too obsessed with making it absolutely perfect. You probably won't be 100 percent happy with your personal statement, but that's okay; as long as on the whole, it reads well, and gets across the main points you want to make, that's great!

As for what to put in your personal statement; that's a tricky thing to give advice on, because personal statements are a very individual thing, and the experiences you have had are not going to be the same as anyone else's. But there are a few things a personal statement will usually include.

A personal statement for medicine will often include: one or a few key reasons for wanting to study medicine, what you got out of your work experience, responsibilities you hold, hobbies and clubs you're part of.

Now, if you're panicking a little, because you're not sure you've 'done enough things' or 'had enough profound life experiences' to write a winning personal statement, don't worry! When I first sat down to write my personal statement, I found it hard to find anything about my life that I could make relevant to medicine other than the fact that I had done GP and hospital-based work experience. But in time, I realised, you can make so many things relevant to medicine if you know how.

In 2014, the General Medical Council (GMC) published a very useful document for aspiring medical students called the "Statement on the core values and attributes needed to study medicine". The document shouldn't be too difficult to find if you search for it online. The statement lists the attributes and skills that are necessary to study medicine. These include:

- **Motivation to study medicine and genuine interest in the medical profession**
- **Insight into your own strengths and weaknesses**
- **The ability to reflect on your own work**
- **Personal organisation**
- Academic ability
- **Problem solving**
- **Dealing with uncertainty**
- **Manage risk and deal effectively with problems**
- **Ability to take responsibility for your own actions**
- **Conscientiousness**
- Insight into your own health

- Effective communication, including reading, writing, listening and speaking
- **Teamwork**
- **Ability to treat people with respect**
- **Resilience and the ability to deal with situations**
- **Empathy and the ability to care for others**
- **Honesty**

These are some of the key skills that you need to show medical schools that you have. Therefore, I would say, it would be a good idea to display as many of these skills and attributes in your personal statement as you can. (The points in bold are the points that I think are most appropriately demonstrated through the medium of a personal statement).

So when you're thinking about the hobbies and activities you do in your life, see if they match up with any of the points from the criteria above. You'll probably find they do. For example, let's say you and your friends play a casual game of netball one weekend a month. That takes organisational skills to book a court and make sure everyone knows where and what time to meet. As a team sport, netball takes teamwork and communication to score goals. Let's say you remember that last month, you got penalised too many times for obstructing your opponent, so this month you're going to be mindful of your movements to avoid that; you have the ability to reflect on your work. So if something as simple as meeting up with your friends to play a bit of sport can demonstrate such a promising number of relevant attributes, I hope you can see that you have a lot more going for you than you may have first thought.

*

Due to the limited amount of characters you have to write your personal statement (the character limit is 4000 including spaces), it is really about quality over quantity. Try to write comprehensively about a few important things, rather than writing really vaguely about too many different things. At the same time, try not to write about things in so much detail that you have room for very few points in your personal statement. If you do this, you run the risk of not expressing enough of the key attributes needed to be a successful medical student. Striking the balance between a good level of detail, and a good number of points can be a little tricky, but give it a few drafts, and you'll get there.

Make sure with all points you make, you explain what you got out of the experience and how it will help you become a good doctor. You might find that a good way to demonstrate your ability to reflect is not necessarily to just rely on writing 'once I reflected on this', but to sort of write your personal statement as one huge reflection on your medical journey up until now.

*

If you're still struggling for personal statement inspiration, I have some questions for you, to get you thinking;

- Do you play a sport, no matter the level; casually with your friends, as part of a club or team, semi-professionally, professionally?
- Do you play an instrument? Do you play in a band or an orchestra? Have you ever composed anything?
- Do you do any volunteering?
- Do you have a part time job?
- Do you hold any responsibilities at school? Sports captain, prefect, school newspaper reporter?

- Have you ever won anything?
- Have you ever been in an emergency situation?
- Have you ever done a group activity or project?
- Have you ever been in charge of something or had to take charge?
- Have you ever been responsible for someone or something?
- Have you ever had to interact with someone and show them compassion and empathy?
- Are you learning, or do you speak another language?
- Do you have an interesting hobby? Anything; chess, reading, drawing, singing, dancing exercising?

*

When going through the application process, both times, I discovered that medical schools can be very interested in your stress management techniques. This makes a lot of sense, as even before you're busy and stressed doctor, the pressure of medical school can burn people out. So it's important that students handle stress well. When I say 'stress management techniques', I don't mean you need to be a fully-fledged psychiatrist with an ongoing self-treatment plan; all medical schools are looking for is that you have something that you do that helps you relax and clear your head. This could be anything from going to the gym a few times a week, to reading a book before you go to bed. The bottom line is, hobbies are great for stress management, so make sure you have one, not just for the application process, but for your entire medical career.

*

So, last but by no means least for this chapter, let's talk about the big question; **why do you want to study medicine?** This is nearly always the first thing people cover in their personal statements and it is also a pretty much guaranteed interview question. It is obviously a very important question to ask yourself if you are making the decision to devote five years of your life to medical school, plus the rest of your life to healthcare. Your answer to this question may determine whether universities offer you a place to study medicine or not. But don't panic! I don't mean you have to write a groundbreaking little paragraph explaining why you want to study medicine, which is more eloquent and compelling than every other applicant's paragraph. I shall explain:

What I found when writing my personal statement was, although I briefly wrote why I wanted to study medicine in my introduction, my personal statement as a whole was a stronger and more authentic answer to this question.

It is hard to be unique when writing your little introductory sentences explaining your reasons for choosing medicine, because most of us want to study medicine for the same sorts of reasons; we want to help people, we want a challenging and varied career, we are interested in the human body, etc.

Because of this, and because of the fact that your full personal statement is how you'll comprehensively answer this question, you can be relatively brief in your introductory sentences and don't need to make your answer crazily unique. Although you should have your explicit answer in your introduction so your personal statement opens well, it's not the most important part of your personal statement. As long as your initial reasons are authentic and personal to you, you should be able to convey enough genuine passion to satisfy the admissions team, even if you think your reasons are going to be very similar to every other applicants'.

Here's an example of the kind of brief answer I am talking about to open your personal statement:

My initial interest in medicine began when I was admitted to hospital for a bizarre headache, and found the 'clinical detective' role of a doctor fascinating. This, paired with my love for human biology, and my passion for helping people, has made me determined to study medicine.

You can go on to clarify and elaborate on things you've mentioned in your opening, using points you make throughout your personal statement. For example, you could say that you learned more about a doctor's 'clinical detective' role during your work experience, and then go on to explain what the doctor did that makes them a 'clinical detective'. So you'll be able to find ways to make your personal statement work without cramming too much into your opening.

Moving onto your 'real' answer; to make sure your overall answer to the 'why do you want to study medicine' question is answered well, I would say, some key things to demonstrate in your personal statement are passion, drive and a realistic understanding of medicine.

Passion: Think about what initially sparked your interest. Perhaps it was an experience like being admitted to hospital, perhaps you have watched medical documentaries, or you've always found the human body interesting. You may have answered this part in your introduction. Read your introduction back and see if it shows that medicine truly excites and interests you.

Drive: You want to show that medicine is something you wholeheartedly intend on pursuing, it's not just something you fantasise about, whilst doing nothing to help make the dream a reality. A good way to demonstrate drive is to explain what you've done to prepare for medical training. Have you read books, watched documentaries, arranged work experience, done an Extended Project Qualification (EPQ), founded a medical society at your school?

A realistic understanding of medicine: make sure everything you write about medicine is accurate and unromanticised. Avoid saying something like you want to be a doctor because you like 'House', because it suggests that you have a glamorised vision of medicine; House has an unrealistically lavish lifestyle and he's actually a pretty terrible doctor; he's arrogant, he's not a team player; process of diagnosis is really random, and on the odd occasion that he visits a patient, the way he talks to them is quite appalling. This isn't the sort of image of a doctor that you want to tell a Medical School you admire.

I would suggest thinking about what you have done to explore the medical world further. This is slightly different to preparing for medical training because you need to focus on what you did to understand what a medical career entails, rather than doing things to prepare for what it entails. This is where those comprehensive work experience notes that you've hopefully made come in. Using the example notes from earlier, you might say in your personal statement that you discovered there is more to medicine that simply treating the illness or injury you see in front of you; you need to look at and treat the patient holistically in order to fulfil your duty of care.

UKCAT

The UK Clinical Aptitude Test (UKCAT) is a computer-based, multiple choice test that many UK medical schools use as part of their admissions process. It is a two hour test that is split into 5 sections; Verbal Reasoning, Quantitative Reasoning, Abstract Reasoning, Decision Making, and Situational Judgement. It is the most common admissions test in the UK. The other admissions tests are the BMAT (which is a less common test, used for Oxbridge and a few other Universities) and the GAMSAT (which is a test for graduate entry medicine). But I didn't take either of these tests so I will only talk about the UKCAT.

To take the test, you register on the UKCAT website (www.ukcat.ac.uk) between early May and mid-September, of the year that you are sending in your medical school application. You then book your test for any date between early July and early October. You can cancel or reschedule your test up to 24 hours before you are due to take the test, but I would advise that you don't do this unless absolutely necessary, for reasons I will explain later on. You take your test at your nearest Pearson Vue Centre (the place where you do your driving theory test), and that's that. As soon as you have finished the test, your results will be printed and handed to you at the front desk. Results are logged by the UKCAT consortium, and after the UCAS deadline, the UKCAT consortium communicate with UCAS to find out which universities you have applied to. They then send your results to which ever universities, out of the ones you have applied for, use the UKCAT as part of their admissions process.

How the UKCAT is scored

4 of the subsections of the UKCAT (Verbal Reasoning, Quantitative Reasoning, Abstract Reasoning, and Decision Making) are scored between 300 and 900. Where 300 is a

pretty poor score, and 900 is the score of a super genius. For each subsection, you are given marks for correct answers and then your total raw mark is converted to the 300 – 900 score system. The average score is about 600, and the score of someone that's likely to get an interview might be around 640-750. But the average score changes each year in a similar way to how grade boundaries for GCSEs and A levels change each year, so it is hard to truly say what a good or a bad score is, so don't take any of these numbers as gospel. You will also get a total score for these 4 sections, which is just your scores in each section added up. It is therefore any score between 1200 and 3600. Situational Judgement is marked differently; you are given a Band between 1 (the best) and 4 (the worst). You will get full marks for correct answers and then partial marks for answers near to the correct answer. The raw marks are then converted to the band system. Again, it's hard to say for certain, but often, Band 1-2 is a good score. Some universities will automatically reject your application if you get a Band 4, but from what I have seen, it's quite difficult to get a Band 4 unless you have absolutely zero common sense.

How universities use your UKCAT results

Each university will use the UKCAT slightly differently. You can have a look on the Medicine admissions pages of each university's website to find out not only if they require the UKCAT, but how they will use your results in the admissions process. The basic reason for universities using the UKCAT is that, because Medicine is such a competitive course, Universities need a way of separating applicants, to decide who gets an interview, as most applicants will have very similar grades and work experience. Some universities will have a cut off score, so anyone with an overall score below the cut off will definitely not be invited to interview. Some universities use a points system, whereby you get a certain amount of points, depending on your overall score, which will be added to points received for grades and other things. Some universities care about specific subsections of the UKCAT, and may have cut off scores for one specific subsection. Some universities only use the UKCAT at the end of the application process, to differentiate between borderline applicants. But in general, the better your UKCAT score, the better your chances of an interview and an offer.

How to prepare for the UKCAT

As the UKCAT isn't something you can really revise for, it is hard to know what to do to make sure you are ready for it. I would say, the best way to prepare for the UKCAT is to do as many practice questions as you can, in the time frame that you will be given to do the questions in the test. This will get you used to how the UKCAT is, and along with hopefully making you a bit less daunted about sitting the test, you should hopefully be able to pick up your own little strategies for answering the questions.

I used an online resource called Medify to prepare for my UKCAT, and I found it to be the best for me. It allowed you to do tonnes of practice questions in the timeframe of the real test, on the computer, in the same format as the real thing. I found this extremely helpful as it meant, when I went into the real test, I knew exactly what to expect and there were no surprises. What I also found great about the resource was that once you'd done a set of practice questions, it would let you go back through them, see which ones you got right and wrong, and it gave you an explanation as to how to get to the right answer. So in a notebook, I wrote down the questions I got wrong, and I wrote a small tutorial for myself on how to get to the write answer. I had dozens of questions for each subsection in my notebook by the end, and it allowed me to really understand what each question was asking of me, so I developed pretty good exam technique.

This worked really well for me, but if you don't think it's for you, there are plenty of other resources out there that you might find handy. Have a look online and see what you think will work best for you. You do have to pay for a lot of the good resources; I had to pay for a membership to use the Medify resource; you have to pay for most of the UKCAT courses; and you have to buy the books that have the practice questions in them. Make sure you read the reviews for everything you look at though; I have heard of people paying hundreds of pounds for courses that they didn't find particularly useful.

I would also say, no matter how you choose to practice, make sure you practice answering questions in the timeframe you would have in the real test. The UKCAT is very fast paced, and the questions are only challenging because of the little time you have to answer them. You might find you are answering questions pretty easily at your own pace, but you will be in for a nasty shock in the real test. So from the get-go, answer questions at the speed of the test so that you develop the exam technique needed to answer speedily in the real thing.

Verbal Reasoning

The Verbal Reasoning section is a bit like a reading comprehension; you are given a few passages and asked questions to assess your ability to evaluate the information you have and determine if you can draw certain conclusions from them. You get a mixture of questions that are usually along the lines of 'which of the following conclusions can be drawn from the passage' or you might be given a statement and have the choice between 'true', 'false', or 'can't tell'. This is a very fast paced section so you need to work on your ability to skim through passages to find only the relevant information.

Quantitative Reasoning

This section is like a mini maths test, but it's less about intricate mathematics and more about problem solving. The maths itself isn't particularly challenging, but what is challenging is answering the questions in the very limited time you have. As the test is multiple choice, you may be able to make some educated guesses and estimations at times. You might find it helpful to look at the answers and eliminate some of the answers you know definitely can't be right, as well.

Abstract Reasoning

Abstract Reasoning is all about identifying patterns in abstract shapes, lines, and dots. This section assesses your ability to evaluate and interpret 'data', and not get distracted by irrelevant 'data'. This section is probably the weirdest and most unlike anything you would have encountered before, but the more practice questions you do, the easier the patterns will be to spot. I made a list of all of the patterns I had ever encountered, and when I did a question, I would go through the list in my head to see if it fitted any of the; most of the time they did.

Decision Making

This section is about using logic, analysing arguments, and analysing statistics to get to a specific conclusion or decision. The material you are given may vary between graphs and tables, diagrams, or short passages, and from them you will have to answer either 'yes or no' questions, or pick one correct answer from a choice of four. You'll need a mix of all the skills used in the first three subsections; the best way to master this subsection is to do as many practice questions as you can and develop good exam technique.

Situational Judgement

In this section, you will be given some scenarios which will contain different ethical issues. You will also be given a list of actions or background factors to rank. You have to rank the actions you could take to deal with the situation from 'Very appropriate' to 'Very Inappropriate'. And you have to rank the background factors that are to be considered before deciding what to do from 'Very Important' to 'Not Important at all'. Although this section may seem like common sense, and in a way, it is, don't neglect this section in your preparations because you think it's going to be an easy section. It's important to get comfortable with the scenarios and what each question is really asking of you.

When to take the test

You can take the test whenever you want, but my advice would be to take it in the summer holidays, before you go back to school and find yourself with a lot more to worry about than just preparing for your UKCAT. I would also advise you take the test towards the end of the holidays, giving yourself plenty of time to prepare. From what I found, a good amount of time to prepare for your UKCAT is about 4 – 5 weeks, with 2-3 weeks of more casual preparation, and then 1-2 weeks of more lengthy and concentrated preparation.

Why you should avoid rescheduling your test

The first year I took the UKCAT, I booked it for the end of August, but I spent the summer holidays doing anything but preparing for the test. I then panicked the day before, and rescheduled my test. But because most people had already booked their tests by that point, there were hardly any available slots, so I ended up taking the test on the last day the UKCAT was available to be sat, in October. This was a disaster as I was trying to prepare for the test, do all of my homework, finish off my personal statement, and work on my Extended Project. So I just became very stressed and unproductive, and I came out a pretty mediocre score. The second time I took the UKCAT, a year later, I was determined not to fall into the same trap, so I booked my test for the end of August, and I refused to reschedule. This forced me to prepare for my test, so I came out with a really good score. So then I had the UKCAT out of the way, giving me over a month to pick my universities and work on my personal statement before the UCAS deadline. So I would say, save yourself the stress and disappointment, and just prepare for your test the first time round.

Why people find the UKCAT intimidating

Everyone that I've ever known who's taken the UKCAT, including myself (both times), has said that before they sat the test, they were probably the most nervous they have ever been. And from what I've worked out, the only reason for this is because the UKCAT is unlike any test anyone has taken before; it's simply fear of the unknown. Yes, the test is incredibly fast paced and a little bit bizarre, but with practice, you will get used to that. Don't worry if you find that you don't have time to answer all of the questions; everyone has to guess the last few, it's just the way it is. Don't panic about the UKCAT; it's two hours of your life and then it's done and you can move on. As long as you do a good amount of preparation beforehand, it will be absolutely fine.

Which Medical Schools?

For most courses, choosing a university is just a matter of deciding which city and course you like the best. But as Medicine is so competitive, you have to be a lot more tactical about your decision. When applying to medical schools through UCAS, you will be allowed to pick four medical schools to apply to. The four you pick should be the four you are most likely to get an offer from, not necessarily the four you like the best. Once you have finished medical school, you are a qualified doctor; that fact doesn't change depending on the university you went to; and you probably won't be a better doctor for having studied at one university compared to another. So you shouldn't worry about how prestigious a medical school is, how big or small it is, where it is, or anything other than whether it is a good match for you based on entry criteria. If you find you're a very good match for more than four universities, then by all means be a bit fussier about which ones you apply to. On the whole, once you've been through the application process and you've received your offers, you can think with your heart a bit more about which university is right for you; but until then, think with your head.

The main things that universities will take into consideration when picking applicants for interview are: Grades, UKCAT, Personal Statement Content, and Work Experience. Each university will put a different weight of importance on each of these things, therefore, it's vital to know which universities care most about which things, so you can apply to ones that care most about the things you are good at. There is lots of information about how each Medical School goes about the selection process online, so be sure to do your research for as many universities as possible! Choosing Medical Schools is something that should definitely be left until you have completed your application; your personal statement should be finished, you should have your UKCAT score, you should have received your most recent set of results, and you should've done all of your work experience. This way, you know exactly what your strengths and weaknesses are, and you can make the most informed decision possible.

The application process, from the medical school's perspective, is basically a process of elimination. Once a Medical School has chosen their interview candidates, they will make offers pretty much based solely on interview performance, as it is assumed that if you got an interview, your application, on paper, was good enough. Therefore, your 'paper application' is only really a means of getting an interview. So, at this point in the application process, the only question you really need to think about is 'Will I get an interview if I apply to this medical school?'

For example, let's say you have good grades, a great UKCAT score, an average personal statement, and average work experience. Applying to a university that cares a lot about what you've put in your personal statement, but only uses the UKCAT at the end of the interview process when deciding between borderline applicants, is not going to be a good option for you, as you are really leaving it to chance as to whether you will get offered an interview. However, applying to a university that doesn't read personal statements to decide who to interview, but does rank applicants according to

UKCAT performance, is going to be a much less risky option for you.

Let's use another example; let's say you have great grades, a low-average UKCAT score, a good personal statement, and average work experience. If you pick a university that has a UKCAT cut off score, or ranks applicants according to UKCAT performance, you could damage your chances at getting an interview. But if you pick a university that ranks applicants according to their grades, has a criteria that personal statements should meet, and doesn't seem too fussed about the UKCAT, your chances of an interview are going to be a lot better.

Interview Style

Nowadays, most medical schools use Multiple Mini Interviews (MMI), but some use the traditional twenty minute interview in front of a panel, and some do a mixture of the two and may include some group work. You'll be able to find information about each medical school's interview style online. Interview Style may be something that you want to take into account when choosing which medical schools you apply to, but I don't think it should play a massive role. The skills used in each different type of interview are nearly all the same, and you probably won't find you absolutely fail at one type of interview, and do extremely well at another type. If you really think that you'll be more uncomfortable doing a certain type of interview, then avoid it if you can. But if you are a very good criteria match for a university that uses a style of interview you aren't keen on, don't rule it out just because of that; you may end up picking a university you're less of a match to, and not even get an interview.

Universities that do not interview - good or bad?

There are very few universities, if any are left, that do not interview. But they are certainly worth a mention in this book as they bring up a good point. Although, the prospect of applying to a medical school and receiving an offer without interview sounds amazing, these medical schools are notoriously difficult to get into and may, in fact, be a waste of an application. To receive an offer from this sort of university, your application must be faultless; your grades must be amazing, your personal statement must be perfect, and your admissions test score must be exceptional. If this is you, then go right ahead and apply to this type of university, it might be the one for you. But this will apply to very few people. Most of us do not have an absolutely perfect application, but that doesn't mean we won't make excellent doctors. In truth, the interview is where you are going to be able to truly shine; until then, the application process, for most people, is just a matter of jumping through hoops; it's about being 'good enough' rather than 'the best'. Your paper application is going to suggest to universities that you are worthy of a place at their medical school, but the interview will give you the opportunity to prove that you are undoubtedly worthy. In my opinion, the Medical School interview is something to 'get pumped' about rather than something to dread.

Interviews

Interviews are the most daunting part of the application process, but having been to five medical school interviews, I can tell you they're not as terrifying as they're made out to be, and with the right preparation, they tend to go pretty smoothly.

As mentioned in the previous chapter, there are a few different styles of interview. There's the traditional panel interview, the multiple mini interview, and there are some other 'panel/MMI hybrids'.

You won't come across too many 'hybrids' as most universities either do MMI or traditional interviews. But they do exist, so just be aware of them. These interviews sometimes involve group discussions, but apart from that they will probably just be a mix of the two more common interview types, so the advice you need for them will be covered.

Traditional Interviews usually last around twenty minutes, and will be in one room, in front of a panel of between two and maybe six people. You will sit in a seat opposite the panel and they will ask you a series of questions for twenty minutes, and then it will be over. It's how you'd expect any regular interview to be. The questions asked in this type of interview will be almost the same as the questions you'll be asked in an MMI, except in a traditional interview, it is less likely (although there is still a chance) that you will be asked to do some role playing, or any written tasks.

Multiple Mini Interviews (MMIs) are so named because you have multiple interviews, and they're mini. You will probably have between 6 and 10 stations at your MMI. A station is usually either; one of many small rooms in a corridor; or one of many cubicles within one large room. The stations are organised in a rough circle or rectangle, so after each station, you'll get up and walk round to the next. Every station will last the same amount of time; usually between 5 and 10 minutes. At each station, you will be asked a question, or will have to complete a task; also there is usually one rest station where you can just relax. You are usually given the question or task before entering each station, and you should get a minute or so to read it before you enter the station.

A lot of people seem to find the idea of MMI's quite daunting – I did before I attended mine – but in my opinion, they are the best type of interview from the point of view of the applicant. There are a few reasons of this:

1. You get time to read the question and think about what you are going to say before you enter the station, instead of feeling obliged to blurt out an answer as soon as you're questioned, even if you don't know what you want to say.
2. If you mess up at one station, you will get marked down for that station alone, which means when you leave that station, you can pretend it never happened and get back on track. If you do well in your other stations, your overall performance is still going to be decent. Whereas, in a traditional interview, messing up on one question may cause the interview to get a little awkward and go downhill. (I've experienced messing up in both types of interview, and it was a lot easier to come back from in the MMI).
3. It's more of an even playing field because all applicants are interviewed by a large number of interviewers, which removes a bit of the subjectivity of an interview i.e. there's less chance of someone getting a place over a better candidate because the better candidate was interviewed by someone who marks more harshly than the person who interviewed other candidate.

So, now you know how the interviews are set out, you'll want to know what sorts of questions you're going to be asked and how to answer them. From my experience, the main types of interview questions are: Questions about You, 'Understanding of the Profession' Questions, Ethics Questions, and Role Play Questions. I will discuss each of these, give you some example questions, and explain how I found each of these question types are best tackled.

Questions about You

These questions are the basic interview questions that give a sense of why you want to study medicine and why you're a suitable candidate. You may be asked to elaborate on things you mentioned in your personal statement, or to give examples of times when you showed a specific skill. To prepare for these questions, make sure you've gone through your personal statement and thought about the different questions they could ask you about what you've written. Some examples of questions you could be asked are:

Why do you want to study Medicine? This question is about displaying your enthusiasm for medicine and showing that your impression of medicine is realistic. Elaborate on the things you mentioned about your decision to apply for medicine, in your personal statement, and talk about the subject with passion and enthusiasm. Talk about what you did to prepare for a career as a doctor and to further develop your interest in medicine. This could be things like doing an Extended Project Qualification, taking on a role in or outside of school that has allowed you to develop key skills or doing extra studies outside school. Make sure to mention what you did to get a realistic insight into the medical world; perhaps you've watched lots of documentaries, or have been a patient yourself; at the very least you will have probably got some good insight from your work experience, so you can talk about that. You also want the interviewer to know that you're interested in medicine for the caring and compassionate side of the role as well as all the scientific and clinical aspects. You need to make sure, within your answer, you are mentioning things you have done in the community or to care for someone else that has brought you a rewarding feeling that you think you will be able to achieve daily in a medical career. For this question, it's better to make sure you have covered all ground, rather than going into lots of detail about one point, so make sure you cover: what sparked you initial interest (e.g. you spent some time in hospital and found the role of a doctor fascinating), what you did to prepare for medicine and develop your interest further (e.g. you did extra studies outside of school about the human body), what you did to gain a realistic insight into medicine (e.g. you did work experience), and your interest in the caring side of the role (e.g. you volunteered at a care home, found the work really rewarding, and now you want a career where you can care for people).

Why do you want to study at *this* medical school? This question will show the interviewer that you have taken the time to look into the medical school, and are genuinely interested at studying at that particular university. Make sure you've been to an open day or looked on the medical school's website, and have a few reasons why you are interested in that university. These reasons can be that you like the city, they have good teaching hospitals, you like the course structure, but it is important to have at least one very specific reason; try to quote something you've read about the university (e.g. it's the best in the country for research into trauma medicine, which is an area of medicine you find fascinating). Otherwise you could be talking about any of the medical schools in the UK and you may not seem as interested or well researched as the interviewer would like.

What did you do on your work experience? This is your chance to use those comprehensive notes from your work experience to demonstrate that you have gained valuable insight into the medical world, and have been able to reflect on your time in the environment. You should very briefly explain what you did (e.g. you shadowed a doctor in your local A&E department) and then describe a case or situation that you came across that taught something important. Don't worry if the cases you've seen are not overly 'dramatic' like a cardiac arrest; those cases are great to talk about if you learned something useful from them; but picking up something subtle from a simple case can be just as impressive, as it can show that you are very observant and reflective, and that you really made the most of your work experience.

For example, let's say you witnessed a doctor talk to a patient about their diagnosis and the treatment they[1] had planned. Then, when the doctor left, you spotted the patient looking unhappy and confused, and then you saw that patient ask the nurse to explain what the doctor had said. So this isn't as 'dramatic' as a cardiac arrest, but this is a big deal to the patient, because they had hoped to have felt more informed and reassured by the doctor, but they were still just as anxious and confused after the doctor had seen them, which would have made them feel even worse about their situation. Being able to pick up on 'smaller things' and understand how much of an impact these things have on patients, is a great skill for a doctor to have and should impress the interviewer. So for this example, you could talk about the importance of communication between the doctor and their patient to avoid making a patient feel more anxious and confused; making sure you use words that the patient will understand instead of complex medical terminology, and asking the patient if they understand or have any questions once you have finished explaining.

If you have time, you could talk about another case you saw that taught you something else, but remember, the interviewer isn't expecting you to say that you learned everything you could possibly need to know to be a perfect doctor, so don't try to cram tonnes of 'lessons' into one case, particularly if they aren't completely relevant. One 'lesson' per case is usually enough, and from that, the interviewer will probably have gathered that you've learned some valuable things on your work experience and that should be enough for them.

What are your hobbies? This is your chance to show the interviewer that you have more going on in your life than school. This is important as you need to show that you are a well-rounded individual. For this question, I would say there are two main aspects you should cover; the stress relief aspect, and the transferable skills aspect. So let's say you play on a volleyball team. You can talk about the fact that you find it a great way to wind down after a stressful day, and it allows you to clear your head. This will show that you have something you do to relax when you are stressed, which is very important for medical students and doctors. You can also talk about the fact that playing on the team has allowed you to develop better communication and teamwork skills which you have been able to utilise during group projects at school; and you can give an example of a conflict you resolved during a group project, with your teamwork and communication skills. You could also mention that you know these skills will be useful as a doctor when working in a multidisciplinary team. This will show the interviewer that you are developing useful skills in your personal life, and you are not only aware of their value, but are able to adapt them for your work life.

What do you do to cope with stress? This question is very direct, so unlike the question above, you don't have the option to go off on tangents, because it will come across as you not answering the question properly. If you're in an MMI and the station is about stress management, talking about transferable skills you got from volleyball won't get you any marks, if anything it could reduce the amount of marks you could ge. So to answer this, talk about anything you do to cope with stress; it doesn't have to be particularly fancy because they are just checking that you can relax, not that you do impressive extra circular activities. You can say something as simple as you sit in your living room and read. You can give an example of how your relaxing activity has helped you in stressful situations. For example, let's say you had an important essay to complete but you kept making mistakes, so you took a break to read your book, and when you returned to your essay you found it much easier to concentrate and completed your essay to a much higher standard than you would have if you didn't take the time to relax.

It says in your personal statement you've done ... tell me more about that. Interviewers are partly looking for proof that your personal statement is accurate. But with this question, they are more interested in giving you the opportunity to show them you have done something interesting, and gained something valuable and relevant to medicine from it. So let's say you've written that you are a school prefect in your personal statement. What the interviewer is looking for is for you to talk about your role and describe a situation where you learned something valuable. For example, maybe you were on duty and came across a younger student, sat alone, crying. You can talk about what you did to comfort that student, and which skills you used by doing this. You can also mention the fact that you learned, as a prefect, you have a lot of responsibility, as younger students look up to you, and the way you act in a situation can affect how a student's wellbeing and confidence, which is something you had never considered before. You can also say this revelation will help you as a doctor as you are aware that even the smallest action by a doctor can have a huge impact on a patient. It is always good to describe something you did well, but it is just as important to talk about what you learned from the situation and perhaps even what you would do better if you had the opportunity again. This will show your ability to reflect which is so important in medicine.

Describe a time you've had to use teamwork/leadership skills to get a task done. This question, is about proving you have key skills and you know how to use them. It is also about reflecting on your actions and identifying what you can do better next time. For this sort of question, you need to briefly explain the situation and your role within the group; you need to explain how you used your skills to overcome an issue within the group; and you then need to explain what you could do differently next time so that things go more smoothly.

What's your biggest weakness? This question is all about reflection and self-awareness, which is so important in medicine. You need to identify your weakness, and describe a situation where your weakness caused problems, and then most importantly, talk about what you are doing to work on your weakness. I would argue that it is a good idea to pick 'typical medical student/doctor weaknesses' such as being a perfectionist, even though others might tell you to avoid being 'cliché'. This is because, you want to avoid weaknesses that are going to be a real problem for you as a doctor, such as a lack of empathy, or poor organisation, as this can cause the interviewer to question whether you are suited to medicine. I don't think it should matter too much if lots of others pick the same weakness as you, it's not about having the most unique weakness. You aren't going to get marked down because your weakness sounded similar to the previous five interviewees. But you will get marked higher if you are able to show perception and reflection on your abilities, and show that you are motivated and able to work on your problem areas. You could also mention, why it is important that you work on your weakness, so that it doesn't hinder your performance as a doctor. For example, if you're a perfectionist, you could say that as a doctor, you are going to have lots of tasks to complete in short periods of time, and so you won't have the opportunity to make sure things are completely perfect or you risk not getting everything you need to do done, which can have a negative impact on the patients that are relying on you to sort things out for them.

What's your biggest strength? This question is similar to the previous one, only the opposite way round. For the same reasons as before, I would say its fine to pick a cliché strength. You still should give an example of a time when your strength allowed you to do something good in a situation; and you should still talk about what you are doing to further develop your strength, as it is important to show that you don't rest on your laurels, and are always looking to improve. You can mention why your strength will serve you well as a doctor, as this will show that you are working out how your current skills are transferable to your future profession. If you want, you can mention why you think you are particularly good at this skill, for example, if you are a good communicator, you can say that you have been part of a theatre group for years and it has helped you with your confidence and interactions with people. This may be a good thing to mention, as it shows an even deeper level of reflection.

Have you ever had to deal with conflict? The correct answer to this question is 'yes', because everyone has dealt with conflict, and if you say no, you're either lying or you won't have the experience to be able to deal with conflict appropriately, when it inevitably comes about in your medical career. Once, you've said 'yes', the important part of this question is to describe the situation of conflict you were part of, and what you, or someone else, did to resolve the issue. You should also talk about what you learned about dealing with conflict from this situation, and what you would do better next time. It is very important to show reflection in this sort of question because these are issues that you are going to face all the time as a doctor, and you need to be able to take something useful away from the difficult situations you find yourself in.

How do you deal with criticism? This question is about showing that you are a reasonable and thick-skinned person, as life as a medical student and doctor is full of criticism, whether it be from colleagues that disagree with how you tackled something, or patients and their families that are unhappy with their care. It is therefore important that you are able to deal with criticism appropriately and constructively. You should express to the interviewer that you appreciate constructive criticism and use it as an opportunity to grow. When it comes to inappropriate, unfair, or non-constructive criticism, you should suggest that you avoid arguments by dealing with the criticism calmly and if appropriate, suggesting to the criticiser that they could have expressed their thoughts in a different way. You could also suggest that you try to think about where the criticiser is coming from to see if you can learn anything from what they are saying. It would be a good idea to give an example of a time you dealt with criticism and what you got out of it.

Are you a follower or a leader? This question is the closest thing to a trick question you should get in your interview. You don't want to commit to being a follower or a leader because you need to show that you can adapt to different situations and take on the role that best suits your skill set. As a doctor, there will be times when you will be the most senior member of staff around, with the most knowledge and experience, so you will need to be able to take the lead, but there will also be times when you will be working alongside more experienced and knowledgeable staff members, and in this situation, it would be more appropriate to take direction from them. So you can see that you need to let the interviewer know that you can do both. You want to suggest that you are one or the other depending on the situation; if you have the most experience and knowledge in a situation, you are able to express that to the others involved, and take the lead, but when you can see that someone else has a more advanced and relevant skill set, you know, and can even suggest to everyone else, that you take direction from that person.

Do you prefer to work on your own or in a team? Like the previous question, you need to explain that it all depends on the situation. If you are alone and are set an individual task, you are very comfortable and competent working alone, but if you are with others and set a group task, you are equally as good at teamwork. You can give examples to back up both scenarios.

What would you do if you didn't get a place at Medical School this year? This question is about testing just how committed to medicine you are. By saying you'd accept that you weren't meant to be a doctor and you'd study biomedicine, or saying it wouldn't matter too much to you because you've got a passion for Art and you'd happily apply to Art School instead; you're giving the impression that becoming a doctor doesn't mean that much to you. Medical Schools are not going to take on students that aren't committed to Medicine because these students are bound to quit when the course gets difficult. So you need to give the impression that a rejection this year will not defeat you. Let them know that you will take a gap year and come back next year, even more motivated to study medicine. But then, the interviewer will still wonder, if you weren't good enough to get an offer this year, why would you be good enough next year? So you need to indicate to them that you are going to reflect on how you performed during this application process; perhaps you'll contact the medical schools you applied to and ask for feedback. And then you'll spend your gap year developing as a person via voluntary work and more work experience, so that next year, you're a stronger candidate. This will show, not only tonnes of motivation, but also that you know what actions to take to achieve your goals.

Understanding the Profession

These questions are about proving that you have a clear and realistic understanding of what the medical field is like, and what the role of a doctor entails. It is also about demonstrating an understanding of key concepts within medicine and why they are important. Some examples of questions you could be asked are:

Why not be a nurse/dentist/physiotherapist/pharmacist etc. instead of a doctor? This question is about making sure you know the specific role of a doctor. You can say that you want to care for people; you want a career where science meets work with people; you are interested in the human body. But an applicant to a nursing, dentistry physiotherapy, or pharmacy degree can say all the same things. So you need to make sure you know what separates a doctor's role from other healthcare roles. Some examples of things that separate doctors from other healthcare roles are: the degree involves very in depth studies of the human body (more in depth than most other healthcare degrees); although doctors often specialise, they generally deal with the whole of the body (unlike a dentist for example); doctors carry out many complex clinical procedures (advanced practice nurses often carry out a lot of clinical procedures to, but often not as many complex ones as doctors); it is a doctor's responsibility to investigate a patient's presenting complaint and diagnose them (this is generally not a main part of any other profession's role). Remember to be very aware of how you are coming across when discussing other professions. Although it won't be your intention, you may find you're talking about a doctor's role with a sense of superiority, and belittling other professions. Many of your interviewers won't be doctors; for example, you might be interviewed by a nurse, and if you're going to tell nurse that you want to study medicine over nursing, you definitely need to do it in the right way! Always be respectful of the other medical professions, and remember that they are equally as vital to patient care as doctors. Choose your words carefully, and if you think that you have said something that may be construed as disrespectful, just clarify what you meant and reiterate that you know the value of the other professions.

What are the negatives of being a doctor? This question is about making sure you're not applying to study medicine because you've romanticised the role in your mind. So, this question is about listing all the negative things about medicine you can think of, even the personal things, because interviewers want to make sure you realise how this career is going to affect your life. You want to mention things like how medicine is a highly stressful career; you will live as a poor student for 5-6 years; you work long unsociable hours, which will not only affect relationships and time spent with your children, but will mean you are almost always tired; doctors get a lot of abuse from patients and their families which is something you wouldn't really get in most other professions; you will witness a lot of destressing things that will really affect you, emotionally; you won't earn a great deal of money in the beginning; you have to take exams all throughout your career, so after all of those long shifts, you'll still need to go home and revise.

Is medicine a science or an art? This is an odd question, but it does come up sometimes. This question is about understanding that medicine is a very unique discipline, in that it doesn't follow a strict set of scientific rules like other more science-based field, because no two patients are ever going to be identical and thus cannot be treated in exactly the same way. But science does play a massive role in medicine. It is how doctors can work out what could be going on inside someone's body to cause a certain problem, and what can be done to correct the problem. At the same time, medicine is far too regimented and scientific to fully be considered an art, and yet there is an art to medicine; there is an art to talking to patients, and an art to spotting patterns or anomalies and forming a diagnosis from these. The answer that the interviewer is looking for is 'a mix of both', but the important part of this question is explaining why this is your answer in a way that expresses that you understand the uniqueness of medicine.

What is the difference between empathy and compassion?
Obviously, empathy and compassion are two key aspects of medicine, but they have similarities that cause people to get the two confused, or treat them as the same thing. It is important to know what these two terms mean so that you know why they are important, and how they can cause issues. That's the main premise for a question like this.

So, empathy is the ability to feel the emotions of another person by putting yourself in their shoes. Whereas, compassion is having sympathy for the suffering of another person. Both are very important for a doctor to be capable of so that they can show the patient that they care (by using compassion to act sympathetically), and so that they know what to say and how to act with a patient (as they can imagine, using empathy, what will make the patient feel more comfortable).

Although empathy and compassion are key for a doctor, if not used appropriately, they can cause problems. For example, if a doctor has too much empathy; that is, if they are unable to stop themselves feeling the pain and sorrow of their patients at a certain point, they will become emotionally drained, and won't be able to switch off when they go home. This will prevent them being able to recharge and return to work with a clear head. They will also find it a lot harder to perform tasks, such as vital procedures, because they will be thinking about how much pain and anxiety the patient must be feeling, at a time when it is more appropriate to be thinking about how to do the procedure in the most quick, efficient, and safe way, in order to minimise the patient's pain and anxiety. Furthermore, if a doctor has too much compassion, they may find themselves getting too involved with patients and crossing professional boundaries.

Should E Cigarettes be encouraged or discouraged? This question is an example of when an interviewer will try to engage your scientific mind, to see if you can think the way a doctor should think. You need to form a balanced argument, and use logic to come up with an answer. It doesn't matter if you aren't very knowledgeable about the topic; think aloud, so the interviewer can see how you use logic to navigate yourself through unfamiliar territory. For this example, you can talk about how E Cigarettes are better than regular cigarettes as they don't contain any of the harmful constituents such as nicotine, ammonia, and arsenic, so in that respect they should be encouraged for smokers as an aid to quit smoking. On the other hand, they are a fairly new invention, so not much research has been done on them, so we don't know much about how harmful the substances in E Cigarettes could be, so in this respect, they should not be encouraged as a precaution.

What problems is the NHS currently facing? This question is about showing the interviewer you are aware of current affairs in the medical world. It's a good idea to read some articles on the BBC Health website once a week, and probably once a day as your interview gets nearer. This will keep you up to date with current affairs, so you have topics to discuss. Good topics to be aware of and to look into are: staff shortages, A&E waiting times (especially during the winter months, which is when your interviews are most likely to be), and a lack of funding for key services.

What could be done to improve the NHS? This question is not only about showing the interviewer you are aware of current affairs, it's about showing that you have the reflective skills to come up with realistic solutions. Good things to think about are ways to reduce expenses and waiting times. The impact of both of these problems is fairly effectively reduced by educating the public. For example, you may have noticed posters in your GP surgery that tell you which healthcare service to use for different levels of sickness (if you have sudden chest pain; you should go to A&E; if you have ear pain; you should go to your GP). These posters help to ensure that resources get used appropriately. Believe it or not, as an A&E healthcare assistant, I saw hundreds of patients come to A&E for completely inappropriate things such as a sore throat, and a stubbed toe. And as a result, resources were used inappropriately, which wastes money, and waiting times were longer because of people that were there unnecessarily.

Ethics Questions

Ethics questions are used to test your understanding of Medical Ethics, and to check that you have a strong enough ethical awareness and insight to be a competent doctor. Before looking at ethics questions, it's important to have knowledge of some key concepts within medical ethics. I will briefly go over these now.

Four Pillars of Medical Ethics

In medical ethics, there are four main principles; Autonomy, Beneficence, Non-Maleficence, and Justice.

Autonomy

Autonomy is a person's right to have control over their life. In medicine, this right is usually exercised during decisions about treatment. Therefore, doctors must get consent from the patient before beginning any procedures; if they do not, the can be charged with assault. An adult, who is considered competent, has the right to the choice of treatment, and the right to refuse treatment. However, no one has the right to demand treatments that their doctor feels would be harmful to the patient or to others. For a person to be considered competent, or to have 'capacity', they must be able to make their own informed decisions, and they must be able to understand the risks and consequences of their decisions. A doctor can work out whether a patient has capacity by talking to them, and working out if the patient fully understands the situation. Things that suggests that a patient has capacity include asking questions, or for clarification about something the doctor has said, and being able to explain what the doctor has told them in their own words. Patients who may not have capacity may include patients with dementia, patients with a severe mental illness, patients that are highly intoxicated, or patients that are unconscious. Children, under the age of 16, are technically considered too young to be have capacity. The responsibility of decision making falls to the parents or legal guardians of these children. However, there is a term in medical law called **Gillick Competence**, which describes a child under 16 who is able to make their own rational decisions and understand the risks of their decisions. If a child under the age of 16 can demonstrate Gillick Competence, they have the right to autonomy, and the responsibility to decision making falls to them instead of their parent or guardian.

Beneficence

Beneficence is the principle that doctors must do their best to act in the best interests of their patient at all times. A patient's autonomy takes precedence over this principle, however, in certain situations, such as an emergency where the patient is unconscious or delirious, the principle of beneficence will supersede.

Non-Maleficence

Non-Maleficence means 'to do no harm', which sounds similar to the principle of beneficence, except it looks at avoiding harm rather than doing what is best. For example, researching the best treatments for a certain condition, and giving a patient that treatment, would be beneficence in practice, as this is what is best for the patient. But giving a treatment that isn't necessarily the best, but definitely won't harm the patient, would be non-maleficence in practice.

Justice

Justice is a principle with a few different parts to it. The first part is legality; if something is against the law, for example, physician assisted suicide, doctors cannot do it. The second part is about fairness to all; if an action is going to benefit one or a small number of people, and disadvantage a much larger group of people, it would be considered an unethical action.

Being Non-Judgemental

It is unethical to allow your own personal opinions or beliefs affect the way you act towards a patient. All patients deserve to be treated objectively, and with respect and compassion. When dealing with ethical scenarios, personal opinions should not come into it as they are irrelevant.

Confidentiality

Confidentiality is another important principle in medical ethics, and it is something that everyone has the right to. It is about keeping information about a patient and their condition between only those who need to know i.e. that patient, and healthcare workers involved in that patient's care. Confidentiality is important in maintaining a bond of trust between a doctor and the patient. However, confidentiality can be broken if: not sharing certain information could lead to serious harm to the patient or to others. You should inform the patient that you have to inform others of their situation, if you are going to break confidentiality. For example, let's say you're a GP and your patient is HIV positive. They have not told anyone that they are HIV positive and are not planning on telling anyone. The patient tells you they plan to sleep with their wife without using protection, and he doesn't plan on informing her of his illness. If you cannot convince the patient to inform his wife, you will need to tell the patient that you must inform her yourself, because you have to act in her best interests and protect her from harm. Breaking confidentiality is also commonly done in cases of child abuse.

Assisted Suicide

Assisted Suicide is the act of deliberately helping someone commit suicide. For example, if a patient with a terminal illness wanted to end their life, and their relative brought them some strong sedatives that they knew the patient would use to commit suicide, the relative would be considered to have assisted in suicide. Assisted Suicide is illegal in the UK.

Euthanasia

There are a few different types of euthanasia, but generally, euthanasia is the act of intentionally ending a person's life, to end their suffering. Euthanasia is illegal in the UK.

Voluntary Euthanasia: where a patient makes a decision to die, and asks for assistance in doing so.

Involuntary Euthanasia: where a patient is not considered competent, for example, they may be unconscious, and so another person makes the decision for the patient to die (often because the patient expressed a wish for their life to be ended in such circumstances at a time when they had capacity).

Passive Euthanasia: Causing a patient's death by withholding or withdrawing life-sustaining treatment. However, passive euthanasia is not the same as withdrawing life-sustaining treatment *in the best interests of the patient*. This is legal, and can be a merciful part of palliative medicine.

Active Euthanasia: Deliberately intervening to cause a patient's death, for example, by giving a lethal injection.

The Slippery Slope

The Slippery Slope is a term used to describe a situation where a small action can initiate a chain reaction that leads to a substantial ethical alteration in society. For example, euthanasia is illegal in the UK. However, if it became acceptable for doctors to help patients die, for a time this might be a good thing for patients that wish to die with dignity and the way they choose, who are physically unable to end their life themselves. However, this would be a difficult thing to police, and it would not be long before doctors began ending the lives of patients they thought would see it as mercy, without their consent. At this point, we would be condoning murder.

*

Ethics questions can be quite tricky to answer but once you understand how they work, they shouldn't be too much of an issue for you. I found there is a bit of a pattern to these questions, and I could generally split them into two categories; 'Action' questions, and 'Issues' questions.

'Action' questions usually give you a scenario and then ask you 'How would you deal with this situation'? Whereas 'Issues' questions will often give you a scenario and ask you 'What issues are raised in this situation'? You want to avoid talking about how you would deal with a situation when you've been asked what the issues raised are, and vice versa. With each type of question, the scenarios you are given may be similar, but what you say in reply is going to vary dramatically.

With 'Issues' questions, you need to think about the four pillars of medical ethics; Autonomy, Beneficence, Non-Maleficence, and Justice; and you need to discuss the issues of the situation from the points of view of each of these pillars.

With 'Action' questions, you need to break down your actions into some key parts; showing empathy, offering a solution, thinking about what might happen next, discussing the consequences of ignoring the situation.

So I'll give you an example question and show you the difference between how to answer an 'Action' question and an 'Issues' question.

You are a GP. A 14 year old girl come to you alone and asks you for the contraceptive pill.

What issues arise here?

With the four pillars of medical ethics in mind;

In terms of justice, it's against the law for anyone under the age of 16 to have sex. Therefore, it is technically wrong to provide contraception to someone who is underage as it could be seen as aiding a crime. If she is having sex with a person over the age of 18, that man can be accused of child abuse as this girl is legally a child. In this situation, it would certainly be wrong to aid child abuse.

However, in terms of Autonomy, if the girl has Gillick Competence, so she's able to understand the risks of having sex at a young age, and the risks of using the contraceptive pill, then she has the right to autonomy. Therefore, she should not be denied the contraceptive pill due to her age.

In terms of Beneficence, it may be in this girl's best interests to be given the contraceptive pill, because she is likely to have sex whether the pill is prescribed to her or not, so to protect her against pregnancy, she should be given the pill.

In terms of Non-maleficence, it is a good idea to give her the pill as it will protect her against pregnancy. Pregnancy at her age could affect her socially, as she may not be in a position to raise a child, her family may turn against her, and those factors, on top of just being pregnant at a young age could affect her mental health. But, another aspect of non-maleficence to think about is to check for any evidence of child abuse, because she may be being forced into sex and asking for contraception as her only shield of harm.

How would you deal with this situation?

Showing Empathy. I would empathise with the girl because she is very brave to come to see her GP alone about a very serious topic at such a young age. She is also probably quite sensible if she is thinking about contraception at her age, even if it is seen as insensible to be having sex at her age.

Offering a solution. I would explain the risks of sex and of taking the pill, and I would explain that the pill doesn't protect against STDs. I would question the girl to determine if she had a full understanding of the situation, the laws, and the risks. I would look for signs of abuse such as bruising, her behaviour, and her reactions to questions about her home life. If I had any reason to think she was being abused, I would let her know that I had to contact social services. I would try to gage whether there was a strong likelihood that the girl would have sex even if I didn't give her the pill, and if I thought there was, I would prescribe her the pill as it would be in her best interests. I would try to persuade her to talk to her parents about her situation as they would be her most likely support unit and could offer her guidance.

What happens next? If the girl is certain she doesn't want to talk to her parents, and if I am confident she has Gillick Competence, she has the right to confidentiality and I would not be able to inform her parents on her behalf. I would reiterate that the pill doesn't protect against STDs and offer advice on types of contraception that do, such as condoms.

Consequences of ignoring the situation. It is important to tackle this situation with care and consideration, because not thinking about her case properly could cause you to deny her the pill due to her age. This could lead to a lot more issues for this girl, such as unwanted pregnancy, which could then lead to further social issues, such as being rejected by her family, or not being able to attend school and get her education and social support. Dismissing her case before properly looking into it could also cause vital issues to be missed, such as child abuse, which would then be left to continue. This could also lead to further problems for this girl, such as a mental health problems, caused by a sense hopelessness and of mistrust in the health sector that she was trying to seek support from.

So that's how I would answer the two different types of ethics question. Here is a short list of example scenarios for you to have a think about.

- You're a doctor on the ward and you notice that another doctor has been making some minor mistakes

recently and doesn't look their normal self. You ask him if he is okay and he tells you his brother is seriously ill. He asks you not to tell anyone, and that the only thing keeping him sane is being busy at work. What issues arise in this situation? How do you deal with this situation?
- You are a medical student, and you see a colleague cheating in an exam. What do you do?
- You are a GP and a patient asks you for an expensive new treatment they've heard about rather than their standard treatment. How do you tackle this situation? What Issues are raised here?
- You are doctor responsible for the care of an 11 year old girl who's family are Jehovah's Witnesses. The girl is severely anaemic and the normal treatment for her condition is a blood transfusion. But, you are aware that this goes against the beliefs of Jehovah's Witnesses. What do you do? What issues are raised here? *Note: just because her family are Jehovah's Witnesses, it doesn't mean that they wouldn't be happy for you to give their child a blood transfusion in this situation, so make sure you mention that you would speak to the family about their thoughts*
- You have a membership to a luxury spa in your area. Only members are allowed access to the facilities of the spa. Your friend is a single mother, and she asks to borrow your membership card so that she can visit the spa. What do you do?
- A young patient dies in your care. How do you handle this situation?
- A terminally ill patient asks you to help them die. What do you do? What issues are raised here?

*

Other Types of Ethics Questions

There are a few ethics questions that don't fit the usual pattern. They are less common but still do pop up. For these questions, you can usually use a mix of techniques from the two different style of questions, or you might find they are more straightforward and you can make up a pretty common sense answer.

Here are some examples of other types of ethics questions:

- Should the UK use an Opt-out Organ Donor System?
- Should self-inflicted illnesses be treated on the NHS?
- What is the difference between euthanasia and assisted suicide?

The main question type that I came across that I thought was a little trickier to tackle, was the 'Which would you pick' question. An example of this type of question might be:

3 patients need a lung transplant; a 35 year old ex-smoker who is a single-mother of three young children; a 78 year old retired doctor; and a 7 year old girl. Only one transplant will be possible, who would you give the transplant to?

This question isn't so much about picking someone; it's about looking at each case carefully, and non-judgementally; and about showing you know you wouldn't make this decision alone. I will give you an example answer so you can see what I mean. I will just mention, in general, you are looking for the person that needs the treatment most urgently, and is likely to get the most years of high quality life out of the treatment. By high quality life, I mean a life where that person is able to do and enjoy things that any other healthy person would be able to.

I would have to assess each case thoroughly and give the transplant to the person in most urgent need of it, and who is most likely to have the most high quality years of life after having it.

When looking at the ex-smoker, 35 year old single mother, it is important not to be judgemental just because her illness is likely to be related to her smoking, and may be considered 'self-inflicted'. However, what is important to look at is whether she is likely to start smoking again after the transplant, and whether it is fair to give her the transplant if she may cause avoidable damage to her new lungs. On the other hand, she may be very much in control of her ex-habit and be highly unlikely to go back to smoking, in which case she should not be ruled out as a potential candidate. There is no information about the state of her health, so it is difficult to assess how urgently she needs a transplant. You could say because she is young, her health state is probably good enough for her to wait a while for her transplant, but there is no information to support this, so the assumption cannot be made. She is a single mother, and so she has children that depend on her, and probably her alone. It could therefore be important to take the children into consideration when assessing this woman, as if she was denied the transplant, and became too unwell to look after them, or passed away, these children would have a very difficult and probably distressing life ahead of them. However, you also have to question whether the fact that this woman is a single mother makes her more deserving of a transplant that someone who is not a single parent.

With the 78 year old retired doctor, you cannot really take into account the fact that he was a doctor and may be considered deserving as he gave his life to helping others. This is because it would be unethical to give preferential treatment. However, some may argue that despite the ethical dilemma, the man deserves the transplant as he has paid his taxes for many years, and has probably saved many lives in his career. On the other hand, some may argue that he has lived the majority of his life by this point, and probably will not live much longer with or without the transplant. Again, there is no information as to the urgency of this case, so this, and his chances of a successful transplant at his age should be evaluated before a decision is made.

When looking at the 7 year old girl, a lot more information would be needed to make a decision. For a healthy 7 year old, they should have many years of good quality life ahead of them. This would probably be a good reason to give this person the transplant. However, healthy 7 year olds do not need lung transplants, so it is likely that this girl has a very serious condition, such as cystic fibrosis. This could mean, their quality of life after the transplant may not be as good as one would have thought, and the years of life they have left are probably significantly fewer than that of a healthy 7 year old. However, there may be another reason for the transplant, such as a serious trauma, and as long as there are no other serious injuries, this girl may have many high quality years of life after the transplant. In both of these cases, this girl would probably be in very urgent need of the transplant, which would be another reason to give her the transplant.

For all of these cases, I would need a lot more information, and I would discuss this situation in great detail with senior members of staff and an ethics committee.

So as you can see, you don't need to give an answer as to who you would pick. However, if the interviewer directly asks you to pick someone after you have given your answer, you should give an answer and your reasons behind your answer. You can pick whoever you want, it is about your opinion, and there are no right or wrong answers.

Roleplay Questions

Roleplay Questions are about testing your communication and social skills, to see if you have basic abilities that can be properly developed throughout your training. For this reason, do not worry about being as good as a real doctor; it's just about proving that you've got potential. People can feel nervous and uncomfortable about doing roleplays, but from my experience, they aren't as awful as people imagine. What I did to make myself feel less awkward was I pretended the situation was real, and the actor was actually the person they were playing. Once I had that mind-set, it wasn't about performing in a certain way; it was just about being myself, and reacting to the other person how I would in a regular conversation. I think if you have this mind-set, it can also help you to come across as more natural and genuine.

My advice for preparing for roleplay scenarios is just to practice as much as you can. I found my best form of practice was when I was working as a Healthcare Assistant because I was able to develop my interpersonal skills and interact with strangers in a more mature and compassionate way. So I would advise that you take on a regular job or voluntary role where you have to talk to strangers a lot, because it will allow you to develop the skills you need without you having to think much about it. You can also practice the more traditional way, by getting your friends, parents, or teachers to practice roleplaying with you. Get feedback from people, or even film yourself to see how you're coming across; this will help you make adjustments to your approach. You can also practice alone; I did a lot of this because you can jump straight into it whenever you feel like it. It is always good to practice in front of a mirror when you're alone, because it allows you to check your eye contact, body language, and facial expressions. Don't worry too much about roleplays; they usually go better than you were expecting. Do some preparation and you'll be fine.

Some examples of role play scenarios you might come across are:

- You're a volunteer at a GP surgery. The GP has asked you to talk to patients in the waiting room before their appointments. You are going to talk to Molly. Find out why she has come to the GP surgery today.
- You're a volunteer at your local A&E department. A man in the waiting room is getting very angry about how long he is having to wait. Go into the waiting room and attempt to calm him down.
- You work in a dress shop. A customer has come to collect her wedding dress for her wedding this weekend. Unfortunately, when the dress was delivered to the shop this morning, you discovered that it had a large rip in it. Break this news to the customer.
- You have accidentally ran over your neighbour's cat. You must now go and explain what has happened to your neighbour.
- Your friend is feeling very stressed about his upcoming exams. Talk to him about how he is feeling.

How to act in a roleplay

You want to act professional, natural, and compassionate. Aim to make the other person feel comfortable with you without crossing boundaries. Good ways to do this are:

- Have positive body language – sit up confidently, with your hands on your lap or by your side. Don't fold your arms as it looks defensive and cold. Don't play with your hair, tap your foot, or fiddle with things, as it can come across either nervous, or uninterested.
- Maintain good eye contact – just give the level of eye contact that you would when having a conversation with your friend; don't look away from them too much, as it can seem as though you're disinterested; and don't stare at them too intensely because you'll make them feel uncomfortable.
- Nod or say "okay" or "hmm" at appropriate times – this shows you're listening to what they are saying without you interrupting their flow.
- Leave room for appropriate silences – don't feel like every moment must be filled with talking. Sometimes, if a person is upset, or in deep thought, they need a moment of silence before they continue. Allowing the silence where it is appropriate is a demonstration of empathy and good social skills.
- Be mindful of your facial expressions – try to keep your face neutral and friendly throughout the roleplay, unless the other person says or does something that calls for a certain response. For example, if a person laughs, or makes a joke, smile back and laugh with them. But try not to ever look horrified. Looking horrified or shocked can come across as being judgemental or unprofessional in a roleplay; especially if the person is telling you about something quite personal. Imagine that you are talking to someone who has just been released from prison and they are expressing how ashamed they are for what they did. If they confide in you that they stabbed someone, and

your jaw drops and you lean away from them; that is going to make that person feel even more ashamed and less likely to open up to you again. This is not what an interviewer wants from you. If someone tells you something quite awful, do your best to keep your shock on the inside, and maintain a neutral face. Respond with an 'okay' or 'I see', to show that you are understanding of the situation, and not judging that person.

Things to say in a roleplay

It's sometimes hard to know what to say to someone in a roleplay, especially if your instructions are quite vague. What you say will ultimately depend on the specific scenario you are given, but I have some general tips for what to say.

For scenarios where you are dealing with a stranger, it is good to start by introducing yourself, explaining your role, and asking permission to talk to the person about whatever you have been instructed to discuss. For example, if your instructions say you are a volunteer at a GP surgery, you could introduce yourself by saying "Hello, my name is …, I am a volunteer here at the surgery. Would it be alright to discuss with you what has brought you in today?" If you don't introduce yourself, you may alarm the person you've come to talk to, and they may feel uncomfortable speaking to you. Imagine if a random man walked over to a patient and started prodding the wound on their leg. Would you be alarmed if you were that patient? What if a man walked over to a patient and said "Hello, I'm Dr Smith, I'll be looking after you today. Would it be alright for me to examine your leg?" Would you feel a lot more comfortable letting the man touch your injured leg, if you were that patient now? Of course, because you know who he is and what he is planning to do. The same principle applies in your roleplay.

Ask open questions to get the conversation going. If we continue with the GP scenario as our example, asking a question like "Are you here to see the doctor today?" will get you either a "yes" or a "no" in response. But, asking a question like "could you tell me a little about what has brought you to the surgery today?" You're much more likely to get a more detailed answer that you can build a conversation upon.

Try not to give your own opinion directly. For example, if someone has told you that they're feeling very anxious and don't know what to do about it, it's not particularly appropriate for you to say "well, I think should do some meditation". This is because you don't want to come across arrogantly, as though you think you know what's best for a person you've never met before. You could phase your response in a way that gives your opinion more subtly. For example, you could say "have you ever thought about trying something like meditation?" This gives a gentle nudge, and also checks if the person has already thought about what you're suggesting.

It is okay to ask more personal questions, if you feel the person is open and comfortable enough to share that information with you. It can sometimes be important to ask more personal questions in order to get to the root of whatever problem has been set in the scenario. Always be polite and respectful when asking more personal questions. You may want to add "if you don't mind my asking" onto the end of your question, or before you ask, you could say "would you mind, if I ask you a more personal question?" to make the person more comfortable and prepared.

Listen very carefully to what the person is saying to you, and be aware of their body language; they may be saying one thing, but something totally different is going on inside their mind. Be aware of 'hidden agendas'. This is when someone is brings up a subject, but the reason for them doing so, is a lot deeper than that person initially lets on. For example, a patient may visit their GP and casually talk about a pain in their chest, and that might seem to be the full story. But when the GP investigates further, they discover that the patient is terrified that they've got a serious heart problem because their brother and their father both died of heart attacks. So in your roleplay, be aware that what the person is doing and saying may have a more serious undertone, and be willing to attempt to explore that. If you have a feeling there might be a hidden agenda, ask questions like "is there anything else going on in your life that has led you to feel this way", this may show the person that you are paying attention to them and might give them the nudge of encouragement they need to share their deeper worries.

For roleplays that aren't set in a medical environment, how to act can play on people's mind even more, because it can be hard to see how what you say and do will show the interviewer that you would make a good doctor. The key is to always be polite, professional, calm and approachable. If you are breaking some bad news to someone, be apologetic, and if appropriate, offer a realistic solution. For example, in the dress shop scenario, you could suggest that your shop has a great alterations team, and given the situation, you could talk to the team about fixing the dress and making it a top priority, free of charge. This is a good solution and it's also fairly realistic, which will demonstrate your problem solving abilities. Offering to have the dress remade may be a not so good solution, as having a whole new dress made and getting it sent into the shop, all before the wedding at the weekend, probably won't be possible.

MMI Tasks

Although, it is likely that a lot of your MMI will be taken up by the question types that have already been discussed, it is important to be aware that universities like to set unpredictable tasks for one or a few of their MMI stations. There is nothing to worry about with these tasks; if you have made it this far through the application process, you probably have the aptitude to do just fine in these stations without any preparation. Because these tasks are quite unpredictable, I don't have any specific advice for them. I will say, keep calm, and think logically. It isn't about completing the task perfectly, it's about doing 'well enough'. Interviews are about looking for people with potential; that can be trained to be excellent, they're not looking for people that are already perfect. So don't be too hard on yourself if you think you could have done better, because the chances are, you did 'well enough'. Even if you think the station went terribly, be mindful that it is only one of many stations, and it probably won't ruin your chances of an offer. I have some examples of some tasks to give you an idea of what sorts of things could be set:

- Read an article and answer questions on it
- Maths and science questions – often medical based, e.g. working with concentrations of drugs

- Watch a video and discuss with the interviewer what you saw – these are often about how people handled the situation so be mindful of things that have gone well and things that could have been handled better.
- Listen to a tape and write down the important information– this can often be in the form of a patient consultation, so in this case, important information would include: gender, age, what the problem is, when the problem started, things that make the problem better or worse, other symptoms, any medication they are currently taking, any long term conditions they have (e.g. diabetes), or any significant health problems in the past (e.g. a heart attack).
- You have to find out how many people in your school follow football, and the percentages of people supporting each team. How would you go about organising this?

General Interview Tips

- Have positive, open body language; sit so your directly facing your interviewer and don't fold your arms.
- Maintain good eye contact to show that you're engaged.
- Dress smartly, but don't get too stressed about finding the perfect outfit because the interviewer cares about what you say, not how you look. Subtle jewellery is okay. Make up is fine as long as it looks professional. When you get an interview, you should be given some information about what is acceptable to wear to your interview, so don't worry.
- To prepare for interviews, I wrote down notes on how I would answer common interview questions and

studied these notes as if I were studying for an exam. I would practice answering the questions in the mirror, or by doing mock interviews with my friends. Find a preparation technique that works for you and try to practice daily as your interview gets nearer.

- Interviewers are never trying to catch you out. If you are asked a weird question, take a second to think about what the interviewer is giving you the opportunity to demonstrate with this question. For example, let's say you've mentioned in your personal statement that you ice skate and the interviewer asks "Is ice skating relevant to medicine?" They're not trying to embarrass you by suggesting you've written something completely random on your personal statement (even though they may sound as though they are). They are giving you the opportunity to stand out from the crowd and explain what skills you have learned from ice skating that will make you a better medical student and doctor.
- Control the interview with what you say. You will often be asked quite vague questions, such as "tell me about your work experience". This is great because it gives you the opportunity to say exactly what you want to say, and demonstrate your best qualities. Let's say your work experience wasn't that great and you didn't get much from it, but you developed some great leadership and interpersonal skills volunteering at a nursery. When answering this question, if you mention that something you learned from your work experience helped you later on when you volunteered at a nursey, the interviewer is probably going to be interested in finding out what happened at the nursery and will ask you more about that.

- Don't be put off by 'opposing' questioning. Particularly when answering an ethics question, an interviewer may offer an opposing argument. This isn't the interviewer suggesting that you're wrong; this is them seeing how you handle other points of view. In this sort of situation, acknowledge the other view point, and possibly elaborate on the other view point to show you have a full understanding of it. But then give an argument against that view point to demonstrate you have strong and well thought out reasons for giving the answer you gave. For example, if you say you would give a 14 year old girl the contraceptive pill, and the interviewer says "but it's against the law for someone under 16 to be having sex, so aren't you committing a crime by giving her the pill?" you can say "I see what you are saying, and technically, I might be, but that doesn't mean it is ethical to refuse the girl the contraceptive pill because …"
- There will always be questions or tasks you weren't anticipating; you can read all the interview books in the world and you'll probably still have a question in your interview that you hadn't thought about. When this happens, don't panic, just think it through and do your best. You have the skills to perform well, just believe in your own abilities!

So that's all my advice for getting into Medical School as an undergraduate in the UK. I hope you found it useful, and feel a lot more informed and confident about the application process!

Good luck with your applications!

Printed in Great Britain
by Amazon